Amyloidosis Cure Guide for Beginners

Advances in Research of Amyloidosis Cure

By

Ashton Rhett

Table of Contents

CHAPTER 1

Advances in Research of Amyloidosis Cure

Genetics and Molecular Mechanisms

In recent years, significant advances have been made in understanding the genetics and molecular mechanisms underlying amyloidosis. These breakthroughs have paved the way for targeted therapies and potential cures for this complex group of diseases. we will explores the role of genetics and molecular mechanisms in amyloidosis and highlights the promising research developments in pursuit of a cure.

1. Genetic Basis of Amyloidosis: a. Hereditary Amyloidosis: Several forms of amyloidosis have a clear genetic component, known as hereditary amyloidosis. These include familial amyloid polyneuropathy (FAP), familial amyloid cardiomyopathy (FAC), and familial leptomeningeal amyloidosis (FLA). These conditions are caused by mutations in specific genes, such as the transthyretin (TTR), apolipoprotein A-I (APOA1), or gelsolin

(GSN) genes. b. Sporadic Amyloidosis: Other forms of amyloidosis, such as AL (light chain) amyloidosis, are considered sporadic and not directly linked to specific genetic mutations. However, genetic variations can influence the susceptibility and progression of sporadic amyloidosis.

2. Role of Mutations in Amyloidogenic Proteins: a. Protein Misfolding: Amyloidosis is characterized by the accumulation of misfolded proteins, which form insoluble fibrils that deposit

in various tissues and organs. Genetic mutations can disrupt the normal folding of proteins, making them prone to aggregation and amyloid formation. b. Transthyretin (TTR) Mutations: Mutations in the TTR gene are a major cause of hereditary amyloidosis. These mutations affect the stability and folding of the transthyretin protein, leading to the formation of amyloid fibrils in tissues, such as the peripheral nerves, heart, and gastrointestinal tract. c. Other Mutated Proteins: Mutations in other proteins, such as apolipoprotein A-I (APOA1), gelsolin (GSN), fibrinogen alpha chain (FGA), and others, can also result in the production of amyloidogenic proteins and subsequent amyloid deposition in different organs.

3. Advances in Genetic Testing and Diagnosis: a. Next-Generation Sequencing: The advent of next-generation sequencing technologies has revolutionized genetic testing for amyloidosis. These techniques enable comprehensive analysis of multiple genes

simultaneously, allowing for efficient identification of disease-causing mutations. b. Pre-symptomatic Testing: Genetic testing can be performed on at-risk individuals to identify mutations associated with hereditary amyloidosis before symptoms manifest. This early detection allows for proactive management and potential intervention strategies.

4. Molecular Mechanisms and Therapeutic Targets: a. Protein Stabilization: Strategies focused on stabilizing mutant proteins

aim to prevent their misfolding and subsequent amyloid formation. Small molecules, such as stabilizers or kinetic stabilizers, can be designed to enhance the structural integrity of the proteins and inhibit their aggregation. b. Clearance of Amyloid Deposits: Developing therapies that enhance the clearance of existing amyloid deposits is a promising avenue. This includes strategies targeting the immune system, such as monoclonal antibodies or immune modulators, to promote the clearance of amyloid fibrils. c. Gene Silencing and Editing: Emerging approaches, such as gene silencing through RNA interference (RNAi) or gene editing using CRISPR-Cas9 technology, hold potential for directly targeting disease-causing genetic mutations. These techniques aim to suppress the production of mutant proteins or correct genetic abnormalities.

5. Clinical Trials and Therapeutic Developments: a. Targeted Therapies: Numerous clinical trials are underway to evaluate the safety and efficacy of

targeted therapies for amyloidosis. These include TTR stabilizers, gene-silencing agents, and immunotherapies designed to clear amyloid deposits. b. Emerging Therapeutic Strategies: Innovative approaches, such as proteostasis regulators, chaperone therapies, and inhibitors of specific enzymes involved in amyloid formation, are being explored in preclinical and early clinical stages. c. Combination Therapies: Combining multiple therapeutic modalities, such as stabilizers with clearance agents or gene-silencing therapies, may offer synergistic effects and improved treatment outcomes.

While the development of a cure for amyloidosis is a complex and ongoing process, advances in genetics and molecular mechanisms have significantly expanded our understanding of the disease and provided new avenues for therapeutic intervention. The growing knowledge of disease-causing mutations, protein misfolding, and amyloid deposition mechanisms is driving the development of targeted therapies and personalized treatment approaches. Ongoing research and clinical trials hold great promise for achieving a cure or long-term disease management strategies for amyloidosis in the near future.

Emerging Therapeutic Strategies

In the quest for a cure for amyloidosis, researchers are exploring a wide range of emerging therapeutic strategies that show promise in targeting the underlying mechanisms of the disease. These innovative approaches aim to prevent or reverse amyloid deposition, improve organ function, and ultimately provide a potential cure for amyloidosis. some of the most exciting emerging therapeutic strategies currently being investigated in the field.

1. Proteostasis Modulation: a. Proteostasis Network: The proteostasis network regulates protein folding, quality control, and clearance within cells. Disruptions in this network contribute to the accumulation of misfolded proteins in amyloidosis. Therapeutic strategies focused on restoring proteostasis aim to rebalance protein

homeostasis and prevent amyloid formation. b. Pharmacological Chaperones: Small molecules, known as pharmacological chaperones, can stabilize misfolded proteins, facilitate their proper folding, and prevent their aggregation into amyloid fibrils. These chaperones can potentially rescue mutated proteins and restore their normal function.

2. Immunotherapies and Antibody-Based Approaches: a. Monoclonal Antibodies: Monoclonal

antibodies designed to specifically target amyloid deposits have shown promise in preclinical and clinical studies. These antibodies can bind to amyloid fibrils, mark them for clearance by the immune system, and potentially halt disease progression. b. Immunomodulatory Therapies: Modulating the immune response holds potential for amyloidosis treatment. Therapies that activate or enhance the immune system's ability to clear amyloid deposits are being explored as potential strategies for disease modification.

3. RNA Interference (RNAi) and Gene Silencing: a. RNAi-Based Therapies: RNA interference (RNAi) is a mechanism that can selectively silence disease-causing genes by targeting and degrading their messenger RNA (mRNA) transcripts. In amyloidosis, RNAi-based therapies can be designed to specifically inhibit the production of mutant proteins responsible for amyloid formation. b. Small Interfering RNA (siRNA) and Antisense Oligonucleotides (ASOs):

siRNAs and ASOs are synthetic molecules that can be delivered to target cells to silence specific genes. These molecules can potentially be used to silence the expression of mutated genes associated with amyloidosis and reduce the production of amyloidogenic proteins.

4. Molecular Tweezers and Aggregation Inhibitors: a. Molecular Tweezers: Molecular tweezers are small molecules designed to bind to amyloidogenic proteins and prevent their aggregation into amyloid fibrils. These molecules can

stabilize the protein structure, inhibit fibril formation, and potentially halt disease progression. b. Aggregation Inhibitors: Various compounds and peptides are being investigated as aggregation inhibitors, aiming to disrupt the process of protein misfolding and subsequent amyloid formation. These inhibitors can potentially prevent the assembly of amyloid fibrils and mitigate disease progression.

5. Gene Editing Technologies: a. CRISPR-Cas9: The revolutionary CRISPR-Cas9 gene editing system

offers the possibility of directly modifying disease-causing genetic mutations associated with amyloidosis. By precisely targeting and editing specific genes, CRISPR-Cas9 technology has the potential to correct genetic abnormalities and prevent the production of amyloidogenic proteins.

6. Combination Therapies: a. Synergistic Approaches: Combining multiple therapeutic strategies, such as targeting protein misfolding, enhancing clearance mechanisms, and modulating immune

responses, may offer synergistic effects and increased efficacy in treating amyloidosis. b. Multi-Targeted Approaches: Given the complexity of amyloidosis, targeting multiple pathways and mechanisms simultaneously could address various aspects of the disease pathology and lead to more comprehensive treatment outcomes.

While these emerging therapeutic strategies hold great promise, it is important to note that many are still in the early stages of development and require further research and clinical validation. However, the rapid progress in understanding the molecular mechanisms of amyloidosis and the availability of advanced technologies is propelling the field forward and increasing the likelihood of finding a cure for this challenging disease. Continued exploration of these emerging therapeutic strategies, along with ongoing clinical trials, will contribute to the development of effective treatments and ultimately the realization of a cure for amyloidosis.

7. Biomarkers and Diagnostic Tools: a. Biomarkers for Early Detection: Developing reliable biomarkers for the early detection of amyloidosis is crucial for timely intervention and effective treatment. Researchers are investigating various biomarkers, such as specific proteins, genetic markers, or imaging techniques, to identify individuals at risk or in the early stages of amyloid deposition. b. Imaging Techniques: Advancements in imaging technologies, such as positron emission

tomography (PET) and magnetic resonance imaging (MRI), offer non-invasive methods to visualize and quantify amyloid deposits. These techniques aid in accurate diagnosis, monitoring disease progression, and evaluating treatment responses.

8. Personalized Medicine Approaches: a. Precision Medicine: The concept of precision medicine involves tailoring treatment strategies to individual patients based on their specific genetic profiles, disease characteristics, and

biomarker information. In amyloidosis, personalized medicine approaches can help identify the most appropriate treatment options and optimize therapeutic outcomes. b. Genotype-Phenotype Correlations: Understanding the relationships between specific genetic mutations and the clinical manifestations of amyloidosis can assist in predicting disease progression, organ involvement, and treatment responses. This knowledge enables personalized management plans for individuals with different subtypes of amyloidosis.

9. Collaborative Research and Global Initiatives: a. Collaborative Efforts: Researchers, clinicians, and patient advocacy groups around the world are collaborating to accelerate the pace of amyloidosis research. These collaborations promote knowledge sharing, data exchange, and joint efforts in clinical trials, ultimately fostering the development of effective treatments and a potential cure. b. Global Initiatives: International

organizations and research consortia focused on amyloidosis, such as the Amyloidosis Research Consortium, are driving collective efforts to advance understanding, improve diagnosis, and develop innovative therapies. These initiatives foster collaboration among experts and streamline resources for more efficient research progress.

10.   Patient Engagement and Advocacy: a. Patient Involvement: Engaging patients in the research and development process ensures that their

perspectives, experiences, and needs are considered. Patient involvement can lead to more patient-centered approaches, improved clinical trial design, and better outcomes for individuals living with amyloidosis. b. Advocacy Organizations: Patient advocacy groups play a crucial role in raising awareness, providing support, and advocating for research funding and access to innovative treatments. These organizations empower patients, amplify their voices, and drive

initiatives for better care
and a potential cure.

The pursuit of a cure for amyloidosis requires a multifaceted approach, combining cutting-edge scientific research, technological advancements, and collaborative efforts among researchers, clinicians, patients, and advocacy groups. The emerging therapeutic strategies, personalized medicine approaches, and global initiatives discussed above hold great promise in advancing the field and bringing us closer to finding a cure for amyloidosis. As research continues to evolve, it is crucial to prioritize investment in scientific discovery, clinical trials, and patient-centered approaches to ultimately achieve the goal of a cure for amyloidosis.

Clinical Trials and Experimental Treatments

Clinical trials play a vital role in advancing our understanding of amyloidosis and exploring potential cures. These trials evaluate the safety and efficacy of novel treatments, including experimental therapies and innovative approaches, with the ultimate goal of finding a cure for amyloidosis. Here are some of the significance of clinical trials and highlights of the experimental treatments being investigated.

1. Importance of Clinical Trials: a. Gathering Evidence: Clinical trials provide critical data on the safety and effectiveness of new treatments. These studies involve rigorous testing in human subjects, allowing researchers to gather evidence to support the development of potential cures. b. Treatment Validation: Clinical trials are essential for validating the effectiveness of

experimental therapies and determining their appropriate use in amyloidosis patients. c. Regulatory Approval: Successful clinical trials provide the foundation for regulatory approval by health authorities, allowing new treatments to be made available to patients.

2. Phases of Clinical Trials: a. Phase 1: Phase 1 trials involve a small number of healthy volunteers or patients and primarily focus on assessing the safety, dosage, and potential side effects of an experimental treatment. b. Phase 2: Phase

2 trials expand the study population to a larger group of patients and aim to assess the treatment's effectiveness and further evaluate its safety. c. Phase 3: Phase 3 trials involve even larger patient populations and compare the new treatment to existing standard treatments or a placebo. These trials provide more comprehensive data on efficacy, safety, and potential benefits compared to current therapies. d. Phase 4: After a treatment receives regulatory approval, phase 4 trials are

conducted to monitor the long-term safety and effectiveness of the approved treatment in a larger patient population.

3. Experimental Treatments in Clinical Trials: a. Targeted Therapies: Various targeted therapies, such as monoclonal antibodies, small molecule inhibitors, and gene-silencing agents, are being evaluated in clinical trials. These therapies aim to specifically address the underlying mechanisms of amyloidosis, including protein misfolding, aggregation, and amyloid

deposition. b. Immunotherapies: Immunotherapeutic approaches, including vaccines and immune modulators, are being investigated to enhance the immune response against amyloid deposits and potentially clear amyloid fibrils from tissues. c. Gene Editing Technologies: CRISPR-Cas9 and other gene-editing tools are being explored in clinical trials to correct disease-causing genetic mutations associated with amyloidosis and prevent the production of amyloidogenic proteins.

d. Combination Therapies: Clinical trials are assessing the potential benefits of combining multiple therapies, such as targeted agents with immunotherapies or gene-silencing approaches. These combination therapies aim to enhance treatment efficacy and address multiple disease pathways simultaneously.

4. Patient Recruitment and Participation: a. Patient Engagement: Active involvement of amyloidosis patients and their caregivers in clinical trials is crucial. Their participation helps

researchers understand the disease's impact and ensures that trial designs consider patient perspectives and preferences. b. Access to Experimental Treatments: Clinical trials provide eligible patients with access to potentially life-changing experimental treatments that are not yet widely available. c. Risks and Benefits: Clinical trial participants receive close medical monitoring and regular evaluations, although there may be associated risks. The potential benefits, such as access to cutting-edge therapies and the opportunity to contribute to scientific knowledge, are weighed against the potential risks.

5. Collaborative Efforts and Global Initiatives: a. Research Networks: Collaboration among research institutions, healthcare organizations, and patient advocacy groups is critical in advancing amyloidosis research. National and international research networks facilitate the sharing of data, resources, and expertise, accelerating

the pace of clinical trials. b. Global Initiatives: International organizations and consortia focused on amyloidosis research, such as the Amyloidosis Research Consortium (ARC), Amyloidosis Foundation, and European Amyloidosis Network (EAN), are actively engaged in fostering collaborative research and promoting clinical trials.

6. Patient-Centric Approach: a. Patient-Reported Outcomes: Clinical trials increasingly incorporate patient-reported outcomes, which assess the impact of

treatment on patients' quality of life and overall well-being. These measures provide valuable insights into the effectiveness of experimental treatments from the patient's perspective. b. Patient Support and Education: Clinical trials involve comprehensive patient support and education, ensuring that participants have a clear understanding of the trial process, potential risks, benefits, and their rights as research participants.

Clinical trials and experimental treatments represent the cutting edge of amyloidosis research, offering hope for a future cure. These trials not only provide opportunities for patients to access potentially life-saving therapies but also contribute to scientific knowledge and pave the way for improved treatment options. By supporting and participating in clinical trials, patients, healthcare providers, and researchers collaborate to advance the understanding and management of amyloidosis, bringing us closer to the goal of finding a cure.

CHAPTER 2

Complementary and Alternative Approaches of Amyloidosis

Herbal Remedies and Supplements

In addition to conventional medical treatments, some individuals with amyloidosis may explore complementary and alternative approaches, including the use of herbal remedies and supplements. These natural interventions are often sought as adjunct therapies to support overall well-being and manage certain symptoms associated with the condition. Some potential use of herbal remedies and supplements in amyloidosis management, providing a comprehensive overview of their benefits, limitations, and considerations.

1. Herbal Remedies: a. Curcumin: Curcumin, a compound found in turmeric, has gained attention for its anti-inflammatory and antioxidant properties. Some studies suggest that curcumin may have potential in reducing

amyloid aggregation and inflammation, which are key factors in amyloidosis pathogenesis. However, more research is needed to determine its effectiveness and optimal dosage. b. Green Tea: Green tea contains polyphenols, particularly epigallocatechin-3-gallate (EGCG), which exhibit antioxidant and anti-inflammatory properties. EGCG has been investigated for its potential in inhibiting amyloid formation and promoting clearance in amyloidosis. While findings are preliminary, green tea consumption may be considered as part of a holistic approach to amyloidosis management.

c. Ginkgo Biloba: Ginkgo biloba extract has been traditionally used for its neuroprotective and anti-inflammatory effects. Some studies suggest that ginkgo biloba may have the potential to inhibit amyloid fibril formation and protect against cognitive decline. However, further research is necessary to establish its efficacy and safety in amyloidosis.

2. Omega-3 Fatty Acids: a. Fish Oil: Omega-3 fatty acids, found in fish oil supplements, have anti-inflammatory properties and may support cardiovascular health. While there is limited research specific to amyloidosis, omega-3 fatty acids may have potential benefits in reducing systemic inflammation and oxidative stress, which are associated with amyloid deposition and tissue damage. Incorporating fish oil into a well-balanced diet may be considered, but consultation with a

healthcare professional is advised.

3. Antioxidant Supplements:
a. Vitamins C and E: Vitamins C and E are potent antioxidants that help neutralize free radicals and protect cells from oxidative damage. While antioxidant supplementation may support overall health, their specific impact on amyloidosis is yet to be determined. It is important to note that high-dose antioxidant supplementation should be approached with caution, as excessive antioxidant levels

can potentially interfere with cellular processes and treatment efficacy.

4. Herbal Supplements and Traditional Medicines: a. Ashwagandha: Ashwagandha, an herb traditionally used in Ayurvedic medicine, is known for its adaptogenic properties and potential anti-inflammatory effects. While there is limited research on its direct impact on amyloidosis, ashwagandha may help promote overall well-being and stress reduction, which can be beneficial in managing amyloidosis-

related symptoms. b. Chinese Herbal Medicine: Traditional Chinese herbal medicine may be explored as a complementary approach to amyloidosis management. Herbal formulations, such as modified Mai Men Dong Tang, have been used to alleviate symptoms and improve quality of life in patients with certain types of amyloidosis. However, individualized formulations and consultations with experienced practitioners are crucial.

5. Limitations and Considerations: a. Limited

Scientific Evidence: It is important to acknowledge that scientific evidence regarding the efficacy and safety of herbal remedies and supplements specifically for amyloidosis is generally limited. Many studies have focused on their effects on general health or in other disease contexts, and their direct impact on amyloidosis remains to be fully elucidated. b. Potential Interactions: Herbal remedies and supplements may interact with prescribed medications, affecting their absorption, metabolism, or effectiveness. It is essential to consult with a healthcare professional before starting any new supplements to ensure they are compatible with the prescribed treatment regimen. c.

Quality and Standardization: The quality and standardization of herbal remedies and supplements vary widely. It is advisable to choose products from reputable manufacturers that adhere to strict quality control measures and have undergone independent testing for purity and potency. d. Individual Variations: Every individual with amyloidosis is unique, and their response to herbal remedies and supplements may vary. What works for one person may not necessarily have the same effect on others. Personalized approaches, based on individual health profiles and medical guidance, are crucial.

while herbal remedies and supplements may be considered as complementary approaches to amyloidosis management, their use should be approached with caution and in consultation with healthcare professionals. It is important to recognize that these natural interventions are not substitutes for conventional medical treatments, but rather adjunct strategies that may support overall well-being and symptom management. Further research is needed to determine the specific benefits, optimal dosages, and potential interactions of herbal remedies and supplements in the context of amyloidosis.

Acupuncture and Traditional Chinese Medicine

Acupuncture and Traditional Chinese Medicine (TCM) are ancient healing practices that have been utilized for thousands of years in the management of various health conditions. As complementary and alternative approaches, acupuncture and TCM may also be explored in the context of amyloidosis. An overview of the potential benefits, principles, and considerations associated with acupuncture and TCM in amyloidosis management.

> 1. Acupuncture: a. Principles: Acupuncture is based on the principles of Traditional Chinese Medicine, which views health as a balance between opposing forces, such as yin and yang, and the flow of vital energy

called Qi (pronounced "chee"). Acupuncture aims to restore the harmonious flow of Qi by inserting thin needles into specific points along the body's meridians, or energy pathways. b. Potential Benefits: Acupuncture is believed to stimulate the body's self-healing mechanisms, promote circulation, and alleviate pain and discomfort. In the context of amyloidosis, acupuncture may help manage symptoms such as pain, fatigue, nausea, and neuropathy, thereby improving overall well-being and quality of life. c. Safety and Considerations: Acupuncture is generally considered safe when performed by trained and licensed practitioners using sterile needles. However, it is crucial to ensure that the acupuncture practitioner is knowledgeable about amyloidosis and works in coordination with the primary healthcare team to tailor the treatment plan to individual needs and considerations.

2. Traditional Chinese Medicine: a. Herbal Formulations: Traditional Chinese Medicine

enhance energy flow, and support overall well-being in individuals with amyloidosis.

3. Individualized Approach: a. TCM Diagnosis: Traditional Chinese Medicine utilizes a unique diagnostic framework that assesses an individual's overall health, considering physical, emotional, and environmental factors. TCM practitioners may evaluate pulse, tongue appearance, and other signs to determine the underlying imbalances and develop personalized treatment plans. b. Integrative

Approach: When considering acupuncture and Traditional Chinese Medicine in the context of amyloidosis, it is essential to approach them as complementary strategies that work alongside conventional medical treatments. Open communication and collaboration between TCM practitioners and the primary healthcare team are crucial to ensure comprehensive and coordinated care.

4. Limitations and Considerations: a. Limited Scientific Evidence: While

acupuncture and Traditional Chinese Medicine have been practiced for centuries, it is important to acknowledge that the scientific evidence specifically in the context of amyloidosis is limited. Most studies have focused on their general benefits or in other disease contexts. More research is needed to establish their specific impact on amyloidosis symptoms and disease progression. b. Individual Variations: As with any therapeutic approach, individual responses to acupuncture and

Traditional Chinese Medicine may vary. It is important to work with qualified practitioners who have experience in treating individuals with amyloidosis and consider the unique characteristics of each patient's condition. c. Safety and Regulation: It is crucial to seek acupuncture treatments and Traditional Chinese Medicine consultations from licensed and experienced practitioners who adhere to safety protocols. Quality control of herbal formulations is also essential to ensure product safety and efficacy.

In summary, acupuncture and Traditional Chinese Medicine can be considered as complementary approaches in amyloidosis management. These practices may provide symptom relief, improve overall well-being, and enhance the quality of life for individuals with amyloidosis. However, it is important to approach these therapies with an open mind, in consultation with healthcare professionals, and as adjunct strategies alongside conventional medical treatments. Collaborative care and communication between TCM practitioners and the primary healthcare team are essential for a comprehensive and integrative approach to amyloidosis management.

Mind-Body Practices

In addition to medical treatments, individuals with amyloidosis may explore complementary and alternative approaches that focus on the connection between the mind and body. Mind-body practices encompass a range of techniques and therapies that promote relaxation, stress reduction, and overall well-being. This section explores the potential benefits and considerations associated with mind-body practices as complementary approaches in amyloidosis management.

1. Meditation: a. Principles: Meditation involves the practice of focusing attention and achieving a heightened state of awareness and mental clarity. Various forms of meditation, such as mindfulness meditation, transcendental meditation, and loving-kindness meditation, can be utilized. b. Potential Benefits: Meditation has been shown to reduce stress, anxiety, and depression, while

promoting emotional well-being and a sense of calm. In the context of amyloidosis, meditation may help individuals cope with the challenges of the condition, enhance emotional resilience, and improve overall quality of life. c. Techniques: Different meditation techniques can be explored, including guided meditation, breath awareness, mantra repetition, or visualization. Finding a technique that resonates with the individual and incorporating it into a regular practice can provide long-term benefits.

2. Yoga: a. Principles: Yoga is a mind-body practice that combines physical postures, breathing exercises, and meditation. It focuses on promoting balance, flexibility, strength, and mental clarity. b. Potential Benefits: Yoga has been shown to reduce stress, improve physical fitness, enhance body awareness, and promote relaxation. In the context of amyloidosis, gentle yoga practices tailored to individual needs can help manage symptoms such as pain, fatigue, and

muscle stiffness, while improving overall well-being. c. Styles: Different styles of yoga exist, including Hatha, Vinyasa, and Restorative yoga. Individuals with amyloidosis should work with experienced instructors who can guide them in adapting poses and movements to accommodate any physical limitations or restrictions.

3. Tai Chi and Qigong: a. Principles: Tai Chi and Qigong are mind-body practices rooted in ancient Chinese traditions. They involve gentle, flowing

movements, coordinated with deep breathing and focused attention. These practices aim to cultivate balance, relaxation, and the flow of vital energy. b. Potential Benefits: Tai Chi and Qigong have been shown to improve balance, coordination, flexibility, and overall physical well-being. They also promote relaxation, reduce stress, and enhance mental clarity. In amyloidosis management, these practices may help individuals manage symptoms, improve mobility, and enhance their overall sense of well-being. c. Instruction and Practice: Learning Tai Chi and Qigong typically involves instruction from experienced teachers who guide participants through the movements and breathing techniques. Practicing regularly and gradually increasing the complexity of movements can provide maximum benefits.

4. Breathing Techniques: a. Breath Awareness: Focusing on the breath and practicing deep, diaphragmatic breathing can help induce a state of

relaxation, reduce stress, and promote a sense of calm. Breathing techniques can be incorporated into daily life and utilized during moments of anxiety or discomfort. b. Pranayama: Pranayama is a yogic practice that involves controlled breathing exercises. Techniques such as alternate nostril breathing, belly breathing, or breath retention can help regulate the nervous system, promote relaxation, and improve overall well-being.

5. Guided Imagery and Visualization: a. Principles:

Guided imagery involves the use of the imagination to create positive mental images and scenarios. Visualization techniques aim to engage the mind in creating a desired outcome or state of well-being. b. Potential Benefits: Guided imagery and visualization can help reduce stress, promote relaxation, and enhance overall well-being. By visualizing healing, positive energy, or desired outcomes, individuals with amyloidosis may experience a sense of empowerment, hope, and improved emotional well-being.

6. Considerations and Safety:
a. Individualization: Mind-body practices should be tailored to individual abilities, limitations, and preferences. It is important to consult with healthcare professionals and experienced instructors who can guide the practice based on the specific needs and considerations of individuals with amyloidosis. b. Integration with Medical Care: Mind-body practices should be seen as complementary approaches that work

alongside conventional medical treatments. Open communication and collaboration between mind-body practitioners and the primary healthcare team are important for comprehensive and coordinated care.

mind-body practices offer a range of complementary approaches that can support individuals with amyloidosis in managing their condition. These practices, including meditation, yoga, Tai Chi, Qigong, breathing techniques, and guided imagery, have the potential to reduce stress, enhance relaxation, improve emotional well-being, and promote overall quality of life. However, it is important to approach these practices with guidance from qualified instructors and in coordination with the primary healthcare team to ensure individual safety, appropriate adaptation of techniques, and integration with medical care.

Integrative Approaches

Integrative approaches refer to the combination of conventional medical treatments with complementary and alternative practices to provide a holistic and comprehensive approach to amyloidosis management. These approaches recognize the importance of addressing not only the physical symptoms but also the emotional, psychological, and social aspects of the condition. This section explores various integrative approaches that individuals with amyloidosis may consider for their overall well-being and quality of life.

1. Mind-Body Medicine: a. Mindfulness-Based Stress Reduction (MBSR): MBSR is a structured program that combines mindfulness meditation, gentle yoga, and group support. It aims to cultivate awareness and acceptance of the present

moment, reduce stress, and enhance overall well-being. MBSR may be beneficial for individuals with amyloidosis in managing stress, anxiety, and improving coping skills. b. Cognitive-Behavioral Therapy (CBT): CBT is a form of psychotherapy that focuses on identifying and changing negative thought patterns and behaviors. It can help individuals with amyloidosis manage anxiety, depression, and improve overall mental well-being by developing effective coping strategies and promoting positive thinking. c. Relaxation Techniques: Integrating relaxation techniques such as progressive muscle relaxation, guided imagery, and deep breathing exercises into daily routines can help individuals with amyloidosis manage stress, reduce anxiety, and promote a sense of calm.

2. Nutritional and Herbal Support: a. Nutritional Counseling: Working with a registered dietitian or nutritionist can help individuals with amyloidosis develop personalized dietary plans that support overall health

and well-being. A nutrient-dense, well-balanced diet can optimize nutrition, manage symptoms, and support the body's natural healing processes. b. Herbal and Nutritional Supplements: Certain herbs and nutritional supplements may offer supportive benefits in amyloidosis management. However, it is crucial to consult with healthcare professionals before incorporating any supplements to ensure their safety, appropriateness, and potential interactions with medications.

3. Energy-Based Therapies: a. Reiki: Reiki is an energy healing practice that involves the gentle laying of hands on or above the body to channel healing energy. It aims to promote relaxation, reduce stress, and support the body's natural healing abilities. Reiki may be used as a complementary approach to alleviate pain, promote relaxation, and enhance overall well-being in individuals with amyloidosis. b. Healing Touch: Healing Touch is a therapy that involves gentle touch or energetic

techniques to balance and support the body's energy field. It aims to promote relaxation, reduce pain, and enhance overall well-being. Healing Touch may be beneficial for individuals with amyloidosis in managing symptoms and improving their quality of life.

4. Supportive Therapies: a. Support Groups: Joining support groups or participating in counseling services can provide individuals with amyloidosis a safe space to share their experiences, receive emotional support,

and gain valuable insights from others facing similar challenges. Support groups can also help individuals cope with the emotional and psychological impact of the condition. b. Art Therapy: Art therapy involves the use of creative processes to express thoughts, emotions, and experiences. It can provide a therapeutic outlet for individuals with amyloidosis to explore their feelings, reduce stress, and enhance self-expression. c. Music Therapy: Music therapy utilizes music and sound to promote relaxation, reduce anxiety, and improve emotional well-being. Engaging in music therapy can provide comfort, support emotional expression, and enhance overall quality of life for individuals with amyloidosis.

5. Collaborative Care: a. Communication and Coordination: Integrative approaches work best when there is open communication and collaboration among the various healthcare professionals involved in the individual's care. This ensures a comprehensive

approach that takes into account all aspects of the condition and tailors the treatment plan to the individual's specific needs.

It is important to note that while these integrative approaches may provide additional support and enhance well-being, they should not replace conventional medical treatments. It is essential to consult with healthcare professionals before incorporating any complementary or alternative practices to ensure their safety, appropriateness, and integration with the overall treatment plan.

CHAPTER 3

Future Directions and Outlook

Advances in Diagnosis and Early Detection

Advances in the diagnosis and early detection of amyloidosis are crucial for improving patient outcomes, facilitating timely interventions, and enhancing the overall management of the disease. some of the recent developments and emerging technologies that show promise in the field of amyloidosis diagnosis.

1. Biomarkers and Imaging Techniques: a. Serum Biomarkers: Researchers are actively investigating the potential of various blood-based biomarkers, such as cardiac troponins, NT-proBNP, and free light chains, as diagnostic indicators and prognostic markers for different types of amyloidosis. These biomarkers can aid in the early detection of disease progression and assist in treatment decision-making. b. Imaging Techniques:

Advanced imaging modalities, including cardiac magnetic resonance imaging (MRI), bone scintigraphy, and positron emission tomography (PET) scans with amyloid-specific tracers, have shown promise in visualizing and characterizing amyloid deposits. These techniques can help in differentiating between different types of amyloidosis and assessing the extent and distribution of amyloid deposition.

2. Genetic Testing and Molecular Profiling: a. Genetic Testing: With the

increasing understanding of the genetic basis of certain types of amyloidosis, genetic testing plays a crucial role in identifying specific gene mutations associated with the disease. Genetic testing allows for early identification of at-risk individuals and can aid in genetic counseling, family screening, and personalized management strategies. b. Molecular Profiling: High-throughput technologies, such as next-generation sequencing, are providing valuable insights into the molecular characteristics of amyloidosis. Molecular profiling allows for the identification of disease-specific gene expression patterns and molecular signatures, facilitating improved diagnosis, subtype classification, and targeted treatment approaches.

3. Non-Invasive Diagnostic Tools: a. Biopsy Alternatives: Traditional tissue biopsy, although still considered the gold standard for definitive diagnosis, can be invasive and associated with certain risks. Non-invasive methods, such as skin

biopsy, salivary gland biopsy, and gastrointestinal endoscopy with biopsy, are being explored as alternative approaches to obtain diagnostic tissue samples with minimal invasiveness and complications. b. Liquid Biopsies: Liquid biopsies involve the analysis of biomarkers, such as circulating tumor DNA (ctDNA) or extracellular vesicles, present in body fluids like blood or urine. These non-invasive approaches have the potential to detect and monitor disease progression, treatment response, and minimal residual disease in amyloidosis patients.

4. Artificial Intelligence and Machine Learning: a. Data Analytics: Artificial intelligence (AI) and machine learning algorithms are being utilized to analyze large datasets, including clinical, imaging, and genomic data, to identify patterns, detect subtle abnormalities, and improve diagnostic accuracy. These technologies have the potential to assist clinicians in making more precise and

timely diagnoses, ultimately leading to improved patient outcomes.

b. Predictive Modeling: AI-driven predictive models can be developed to assess disease progression, predict treatment response, and identify individuals at higher risk of developing amyloidosis. These models can aid in early intervention, personalized treatment planning, and proactive monitoring of disease progression.

Precision Medicine and Personalized Treatments

The concept of precision medicine aims to tailor medical interventions and treatments to individual patients based on their unique characteristics, including genetic makeup, disease subtype, and clinical parameters. In the context of amyloidosis, precision medicine holds great promise for optimizing treatment strategies, improving patient outcomes, and providing personalized care.
some of the future directions and potential advancements in precision medicine for amyloidosis.

1. Targeted Therapies: a. Disease-Specific Targets: As our understanding of the molecular mechanisms underlying different types of amyloidosis improves, targeted therapies can be developed to inhibit or reverse the abnormal protein aggregation process. This approach involves designing drugs that specifically target the pathogenic proteins or the underlying genetic mutations responsible for amyloidosis. b. Immunotherapies: Immunotherapeutic strategies, such as

monoclonal antibodies, are being investigated as potential treatments for amyloidosis. These antibodies can bind to and remove amyloid deposits, prevent further protein aggregation, or modulate the immune response to target the underlying disease process.

2. Gene Therapy and Gene Editing: a. Gene Therapy: Gene therapy involves the delivery of therapeutic genes to target cells or tissues to correct genetic defects or modulate disease processes. In the context of amyloidosis, gene therapy

approaches may aim to replace or silence the mutant gene responsible for abnormal protein production or enhance the expression of protective genes. b. Gene Editing: Gene editing technologies, such as CRISPR-Cas9, offer the potential to precisely modify disease-causing genes in vivo. These technologies hold promise for correcting genetic mutations underlying certain types of amyloidosis, potentially offering a curative approach.

3. Pharmacogenomics and Drug Response Prediction: a. Pharmacogenomics: Pharmacogenomic studies investigate the relationship between an individual's genetic profile and their response to medications. By identifying genetic variants that influence drug metabolism, efficacy, or adverse effects, pharmacogenomics can help optimize medication selection and dosing for individuals with amyloidosis, reducing the risk of adverse reactions and improving treatment outcomes. b. Drug

Response Prediction: Integrating genomic data, clinical parameters, and machine learning algorithms can enable the development of predictive models to anticipate individual responses to specific treatments. These models can help guide treatment decisions and facilitate personalized therapeutic approaches for amyloidosis patients.

4. Clinical Trials and Research Initiatives: a. Collaborative Efforts: Continued collaboration among researchers, clinicians, and

pharmaceutical companies is vital for advancing the field of amyloidosis research and accelerating the development of new treatments. Collaborative platforms and networks enable the sharing of data, resources, and expertise, fostering innovation and streamlining the clinical trial process. b. Innovative Trial Designs: The use of adaptive trial designs, basket trials, and master protocols can enhance the efficiency and effectiveness of clinical trials for amyloidosis. These designs allow for the evaluation of multiple treatments simultaneously, inclusion of biomarker-driven endpoints, and the ability to adapt the trial based on emerging data.

5. Patient Empowerment and Participation: a. Patient Engagement: Empowering patients with amyloidosis to actively participate in their treatment decisions and research initiatives can contribute to improved outcomes. Patient engagement initiatives, such as patient-centered research, patient advocacy groups, and shared decision-making, ensure

that the patient's perspective and preferences are integrated into the development and evaluation of new treatments.

advances in the diagnosis and early detection of amyloidosis, coupled with the development of precision medicine approaches, hold significant promise for the future of amyloidosis management. The use of biomarkers, imaging techniques, genetic testing, non-invasive diagnostic tools, artificial intelligence, and machine learning are advancing the field, enabling early and accurate diagnosis. Meanwhile, precision medicine approaches, including targeted therapies, immunotherapies, gene therapy, pharmacogenomics, and personalized treatment strategies, are revolutionizing treatment approaches, aiming to improve patient outcomes and quality of life. Continued research, collaboration, and patient engagement are crucial for further advancements in these areas, paving the way for a more personalized and effective approach to amyloidosis care.

CHAPTER 4

Hope for a Cure: The Road Ahead

Amyloidosis is a complex and challenging disease, but advancements in research and treatment approaches provide hope for a cure in the future. the ongoing efforts and future directions in the quest for a cure for amyloidosis.

1. Enhanced Understanding of Disease Mechanisms: a. Molecular Pathways: Continued research is focused on unraveling the intricate molecular pathways involved in amyloidosis. By deepening our understanding of the underlying mechanisms, researchers can identify new targets for therapeutic intervention and develop more effective treatments. b. Proteostasis Network: Investigating the proteostasis network, which regulates protein folding,

quality control, and clearance, can provide insights into the dysregulation that occurs in amyloidosis. Understanding the interplay between different components of this network may lead to innovative strategies to restore protein homeostasis and prevent amyloid deposition.

2. Novel Therapeutic Approaches: a. Small Molecule Inhibitors: Development of small molecule inhibitors that can disrupt the formation or aggregation of amyloid fibrils is an active area of

research. These inhibitors may target specific steps in the amyloid cascade, preventing the accumulation of misfolded proteins and subsequent tissue damage. b. Immunotherapies: Advancements in immunotherapy approaches, such as monoclonal antibodies and immune modulators, offer promise in targeting and clearing amyloid deposits. These therapies can help halt disease progression and potentially reverse amyloidosis-related organ damage. c. Gene Editing and Gene Therapy: Gene editing technologies, including CRISPR-Cas9, hold the potential to correct disease-causing genetic mutations, while gene therapy approaches can provide a means to deliver therapeutic genes to affected tissues. These approaches offer a curative potential by addressing the root genetic causes of amyloidosis.

3. Regenerative Medicine and Tissue Engineering: a. Stem Cell Therapies: Stem cell transplantation and regenerative medicine approaches hold promise in

restoring damaged tissues affected by amyloid deposition. Stem cells can differentiate into specific cell types and replace the dysfunctional or damaged cells, promoting tissue repair and regeneration. b. Tissue Engineering: Tissue engineering aims to create functional, artificial tissues that can replace damaged or lost tissues affected by amyloidosis. By combining biomaterials, cells, and bioactive molecules, tissue-engineered constructs can offer potential solutions for organ restoration and repair.

4. Collaborative Research Initiatives: a. International Collaborations: International collaborations and research networks play a critical role in advancing amyloidosis research. By fostering the exchange of knowledge, sharing of resources, and harmonization of efforts, these collaborations accelerate progress towards understanding the disease and developing effective treatments. b. Patient Registry Networks: The establishment of patient registry networks allows for the collection and analysis

of data from a large number of amyloidosis patients. These registries facilitate research, aid in clinical trial recruitment, and enable better characterization of disease subtypes and outcomes.

5. Advocacy and Awareness:
a. Increased Funding: Advocacy efforts aimed at raising awareness about amyloidosis can help secure increased funding for research and clinical trials. Adequate funding is essential for driving innovation, attracting top researchers, and expediting the development of new

treatments and potential cures. b. Patient Support: Patient support organizations and advocacy groups play a vital role in providing resources, education, and a platform for patients and caregivers to share experiences and support one another. These organizations contribute to the overall well-being of individuals with amyloidosis and promote a sense of community.

While the road to a cure for amyloidosis may be challenging, the ongoing research efforts, technological advancements, and collaborative initiatives provide hope for significant progress in the coming years. With a multifaceted approach that combines enhanced understanding of disease mechanisms, novel therapeutic strategies, regenerative medicine, collaborative research, and increased awareness, the goal of finding a cure for amyloidosis becomes increasingly attainable. By continuing to push the boundaries of scientific knowledge, advocating for increased research funding, and prioritizing patient-centric approaches, we move closer to a future where amyloidosis can be effectively treated or even prevented, offering renewed hope and improved quality of life for individuals affected by this debilitating condition.

www.ingramcontent.com/pod-product-compliance
Lightning Source LLC
Chambersburg PA
CBHW051819250726
48659CB00005B/1560